C000058019

THE PATIENT'S GUIDE TO: COLORECTAL CANCER

*Frequently asked questions
answered by surgeons*

Marco Sorgi Venturoni
Cristopher Varela Moreno
Adrián Terán Cardoza

ISBN: 9798655452640
Imprint: Independently published

On the cover:
Photograph by Maria Cecilia Peña, taken in the operating rooms of the Leopoldo Aguerrevere Maternity and Clinical Center, Caracas, Venezuela.
Surgeons: Marco Sorgi, Adrián Terán, and Cristopher Varela. Anesthesiologist: Eduardo Perera.

Copy Editor: Alessandro V. Bifolco De Sena

CONTENTS

ABOUT THE AUTHORS

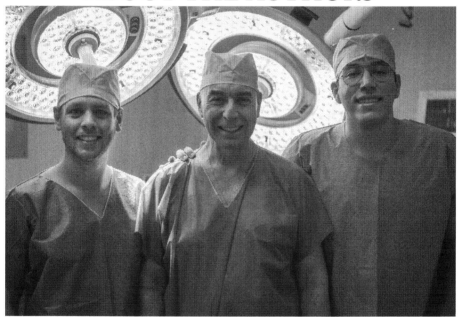

Marco Sorgi-Venturoni

Medical Surgeon graduated from Universidad Central de Venezuela (1972). General Surgeon (1977). Digestive Tract Surgeon Birmingham UK (1983). Medical Doctor - Birmingham UK (1983). Grassi Award from the Digestive Surgical Society - Tokyo (1982). Armchair Number Individual III National Academy of Medicine of Venezuela. Founding Member of the Venezuelan Society of Coloproctology (1987) and President (2005-2008)."Commendatore della Repubblica" honor awarded by the Republic of Italy (2005) for its humanitarian activities in Venezuela.

Cristopher Varela-Moreno

Medical Surgeon graduated from Universidad de Carabobo - Venezuela (2013). General Surgeon - Universidad Central de Venezuela (2017). Coloproctology Hospital Domingo Luciani (2019). Alberto Ferrer Award - Sociedad Venezolana de Cirugía (2018). Student of the Doctorate in Health Sciences. Universidad Central de Venezuela.

Adrián Terán-Cardoza

Medical Surgeon graduated from Universidad Rómulo Gallegos - Venezuela (2012). General Surgeon - Universidad Central de Venezuela (2017). Coloproctology Hospital Domingo Luciani (2019). Alberto Ferrer Award - Sociedad Venezolana de Cirugía (2018). Student of the Doctorate in Health Sciences. Universidad Central de Venezuela.

ABOUT THIS BOOK

It is comforting to see in this work "The Patients Guide to Color-ectal Cancer" a less fatalistic view of what the message of having cancer means. It is aimed as a kind source of knowledge to the patient and his relatives. Therein lies the value of writing to involve families in a situation that generates a catastrophic notification like this, that may unravel the most stable bases of an individual's personality and that transports them, their family and community. Today this diagnosis is still taken inexorably with the same fatalistic and terminal vision of a hundred years ago, regardless of modern times and the greatest diagnostic resources, nanotechnologies, innovative diagnostic therapies and communications without intermediaries that promote social networks. But, this work puts in the hands of patients and families an extraordinary tool that simplifies this path that begins with an appointment scheduled by the coloproctologist who confronts him face to face with his reality. Here we find the simplest answers to the most common questions that patients ask spontaneously to their treating physicians in the phases of assimilation of the problem, their diagnostic qualification process and finally those of both surgical and medical oncology treatment.

We believe that this book must become a must-read publication in order to achieve a comprehensive understanding of this pathology, where the burden so difficult to assume is sought to be distributed equally among specialist doctors, patients and their entire family and community. An expression of team work that aims to involve many in a problem that was previously only seen by a single individual.

Enrique López-Loyo

Chair XXXI

National Academy of Medicine, Venezuela

PROLOGUE

"You are not going to die from this"

That was the phrase of Dr. Cono Gumina when, in front of a screen, he showed me a tumor occupying approximately 60% of the colon's lumen.

He didn't give me time to worry.

I didn't go to the clinic because I suspected colon cancer. I went there to check my stomach, and in fact, I was diagnosed with chronic gastritis.

But Dr. Gumina further suggested doing a colonoscopy, enough proof to condemn me to the treatment that started soon after.

But his opening sentence kept uncertainty away from taking over my mind.

If I am not going to die, why should I worry?

However, there is a risk. The statistics that will be presented to you in this book, and the information that you will get about the chances of getting colon cancer may make you decide to have a colonoscopy.

And to take better care of yourself, in general.

Being a cancer patient taught me not to believe in "iron health." Despite having healthy habits, and I mean eating a little bit of everything and lots of vegetables and fruits (not for health or fashion, but because I like it!), My body grew that tumor, which nowadays I have no interest in getting to know how it formed.

The alcohol? Well ... I am Venezuelan, and I suffer from that ingrained habit of the Venezuelan public to think that a humorist with alcohol will always be funnier.

It is not easy to get sick from the colon. The condition of a colostomy was, to me, the most challenging part of the treatment. Those were 7 long months.

It is necessary to add that chemotherapies, radiotherapies, surgeries, and more chemotherapies were also unpleasant and changed my way of life. But the guidance and advice of Dr. Carlos Canela, who decided the oncologic part of the treatment, helped me to cope with this stage.

Then, Dr. Armando Gil's surgical intervention did the curative part.

I was not lucky enough to have read a book like this. I had to compare observations on the subject obtained from my doctors and the internet. However, it allowed me and my relatives to learn about something we would not have been interested in if I had not gotten the disease.

But I am very sure that this book will change and educate readers, so that they have accurate information and discover all forms of action to combat such a situation.

It is written with the authority and experience that has built the fame of Venezuelan medicine: always correct, always professional, and still very human.

Cheers to Venezuelan Doctors and their ability to heal with love, and always smiling!

Emilio Lovera

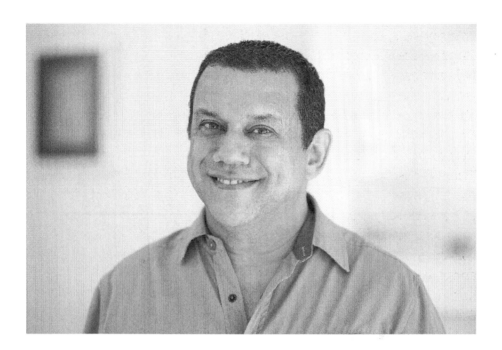

Emilio Lovera is a Venezuelan voice actor and humorist with 40 years of an artistic career. Internationally recognized for his participation in successful theater, radio, and television productions.

FOREWORD

It is no secret that the doctor-patient relationship is an essential factor in medical practice.

It seems to me —and it's a very personal point of vie — that medicine is one of the professions closest to God. Their conduct is full of attitudes and values that provide them an almost divine character. Those who met Dr. José Gregorio Hernández, our dear Venezuelan venerable, say so.

Fortunately, I have doctors whose professional and humanitarian attitudes exceed the expectations of any patient. Kindness, wisdom, and bonhomie are part of what they have shown me.

Here we have a trio of "medical gentlemen," with extraordinary human virtues, and who I am also honored to be their patient: doctors Marcos Sorgi, Cristopher Varela, and Adrián Terán.

They are colorectal surgeons, that means specialists in colon, rectum, and anus. They have been kind enough to write this beautiful text where they provide us with knowledge in a simple language, easy to read and understand, to discern and prevent Colon cancer. And it comes with an added value: It is not only aimed at patients, but also at family members, and anyone interested in quality reading on the subject.

The contribution and usefulness of this work is invaluable. We have all known someone who has or has had colon cancer, or worse, we have it within our family.

In my case, I had an uncle: Angel, who passed away a year ago as a victim of this condition. I am sure that if he had had an orientation like the one described in this text, perhaps his ailment would have been more comfortable and maybe, he would still be with us.

This book is written in the first person, from the patient's perspective, with the simple and common questions that we all ask, so that we can understand it. It is the fundamental objective of its authors, that we become aware of the responsibility that we all have for the care and prevention of this disease.

You will find professional advice for body medicine here. Still, there are also two collaborative chapters dedicated to medicine for the soul because we are an indissoluble whole.

This work summarizes part of Dr. Sorgi, accompanied by the youth, passion, and desire of Cristopher and Adrián so that you and I, reader friend, take care, love, and become aware of that vital part of our body called the colon.

To me, it is an honor to invite you to share this excellent reading.

Ana Finol

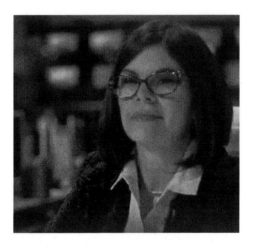

Ana Finol is responsible for the planning and execution of the different newsreels, advances, summaries and special reports of one of the main television channels in Venezuela and the only 24-hour news channel in the country.

CHAPTER I:

* * *

What's going on?

DO I HAVE CANCER?

We've heard the word "cancer" and identify it for some unconscious reason with "suffering" and "death." We always think that it is something that happens to another person. We never wonder: could I have cancer? The truth is that none of us is prepared to face this possibility.

We always think "cancer" is something that could happen to others, but never to us! Fear causes us to block our thoughts from a shocking reality forgetting it can affect us all equally.

Cancer is a disease that causes us high levels of anxiety and uncertainty. It may cause terrible fear and hopelessness, mainly because we do not have proper guidance to help us understand what we face.

What to do? Where to go? Who could help me? How do I confirm it? Could the doctor be wrong? Is there a cure? Many questions arise in this unexpected situation. Cancer not visible to the naked eye, such as colorectal cancer, produces even more uncertainty.

The World Health Organization (WHO) is an expert in collecting figures, statistics, and interpreting their results. According to their information, cancer represents the second cause of death worldwide, with more than 9.6 million deaths per year.

World statistics indicate that colorectal cancer ranks third in order of frequency, with about 800 thousand deaths per year. The bad news is that it is not visible as it develops deep in the colon or rectum. It has few symptoms at the beginning; most of the time, when it is diagnosed, it is already in an advanced stage of the disease.

The onset of colorectal cancer occurs more frequently between 45 and 70 years of age. However, in recent years, it has been detected in younger and younger people more regularly.

Colorectal cancer is the fourth most common cancer in the Americas. More than 240,000 new cases are diagnosed each year in the region, and approximately 112,000 deaths occur annually due to this disease.

In the United States alone, the figures are around 140,000 new cases per year, and it is expected that, by 2030, new cases will increase by 60% if prevention measures are not taken.

In the European Union, the incidence is estimated at 357 thousand new cases per year, which represents about 15 to 25 cases per 100,000 inhabitants, and an increase in both sexes is also expected in the future. What do these numbers mean to us? How can these numbers affect my loved ones or me? Am I really at risk of having colon or rectal cancer?

We can say that if we attend a concert with 100,000 people, there will be between 2 and 4 spectators with colorectal cancer in the public who may not yet know it. Now, if it's a stranger, I probably don't care much, but what if one of those spectators were to be me?

That is why, based on general statistics, to the initial question of "Could I have colorectal cancer?" The answer would be: "Yes, it is possible," especially if you have risk factors to develop the disease.

The American Cancer Association estimates that colorectal cancer accounts for at least 8% of cancer deaths. In Europe, mortality is between 4 and 10 per 100,000 inhabitants per year. The good news is that the number of deaths due to this cause has decreased over the past two decades due to technological advances to improve the diagnosis and the development of new and increasingly better treatment therapies that have allowed improving the survival rates of patients

At this time, 6 out of 10 people who have had colorectal cancer are alive 5 years after initial diagnosis and receive adequate treatment. Even better, for patients diagnosed in the early stages of the disease, this survival rate amounts to 8 out of 10.

Unfortunately, only a minority of people are diagnosed early, many times because they are afraid to consult a doctor, insecurity, or disbelief to accept this possibility. In fact, many patients visit in advanced stages of the disease due to the intensification of symptoms, which considerably reduces their chances of cure.

WHY ME?

If you are over 40 years old, you have fed yourself with processed foods, you eat a lot of red meat, and you live with worries: you have high-risk factors.

The incidence of colorectal cancer has decreased in the past two decades, mainly due to new significant disease knowledge by doctors and patients of risk factors and the advances in research and diagnostic methods.

Between 2005 and 2014, the presence of colorectal cancer decreased by approximately 4% for adults over 55 years. However, it increased by almost 3% for those under 55 and even practically 2% in young adults.

According to statements by the World Health Organization (WHO), between 30% and 50% of cancers can be avoided, and colorectal cancer is no exception. For this, we must try to reduce the risk factors and apply preventive strategies based on the scientific knowledge of this pathology.

If we diagnose it early and treat it in time, the chances of recovery for many types of cancer are excellent.

The late diagnosis of the disease considerably reduces the possibility of a cure. It decreases life expectancy to about 2 in 10 people in the first 5 years. Therefore, the sooner the diagnosis is established, the more likely it is for the total cure and long-term survival, now:

How do I prevent colorectal cancer?

How can I take care of myself and my relatives?

Am I at a higher risk of having it than other people?

It is necessary to instruct us a little about essential topics, for example: Where does cancer come from?

Cancer is caused by the transformation of healthy cells to tumor cells in a multi-stage process that usually consists of the progression of a precancerous lesion to a malignant tumor.

These alterations are the result of the interaction between the genetic factors of the patient and the external environmental factors, the latter are preventable and/or modifiable.

The leading resource we have to reduce the possibility of developing colorectal cancer is preventing modifiable risk factors. For example: changing our lifestyle, avoiding overweight, and improving nutrition are tools to reduce the incidence of this disease.

Today it is known that the consumption of tobacco and alcohol, a poor diet, and sedentarism are the main risk factors related to the development of cancer in general. Smoking alone leads to 22% of cancer deaths worldwide and is, by itself, the most critical risk factor.

Similarly, the consumption of fats and red meat, as well as being overweight, are directly related to the development of colorectal cancer.

Likewise, low consumption of water and fiber are associated with chronic constipation, which determines the permanence of the feces in the colonic tract and constant trauma of the intestinal mucosa.

Aging is a factor associated with the onset of cancer. Probably, because risk factors accumulate over time; also, a progression of age is combined with the loss of effectiveness of cell repair mechanisms. For this reason, elderly patients should be more attentive to the signs and symptoms of the disease and go to the doctor at the slightest suspicion. For the very elderly, family members are a determining factor because they must be the ones to recognize changes or symptoms that suggest they should be studied.

Although there are genetic factors associated with the development of colorectal cancer, 75% of cases of colon and rectal cancer may not depend on this. This means that of every 10 people who develop this disease, approximately 7 had the same probability of suffering from it. Only 3 of them are associated with inheritance factors.

The development of studies on human genetic map is going to make more precise every day to anticipate increased possibilities of developing colon cancer. This type of research of genetic maps is pretty advanced for the prediction of breast and gynecological cancer.

However, people with a family history of colorectal cancer are twice as likely to suffer from this disease than the general population, regardless of whether or not they avoid modifiable risk factors. This risk increases up to 4 times if there are several family members affected. It might be even higher if one of them was diagnosed before age 45 or if they are first-line relatives such as mom, dad, or siblings.

Likewise, if you have had a history of adenomatous polyps, especially if they are large, multiple, or, if any, show dysplasia, you might have a higher risk of suffering from colorectal cancer.

The same happens if you suffer from inflammatory bowel diseases such as ulcerative rectocolitis or Crohn's disease. Therefore, evaluations should be done at an earlier age due to the relationship of these disorders with colorectal cancer.

Is the development of colorectal cancer really linked randomly? Is it a fortuitous event? The development of cancer is closely related to inhibited emotions, sorrows, and deep resentments. Some of them very old concerning something or a situation that disturbs us in the present and to which we never dared to express those deep feelings.

Even though cancer can occur after a personal tragedy, a painful divorce, loss of employment, loss of a loved one, or other emotional impacts usually results in years of internal conflict, sorrows, grudges, hatred, confusion, and tension.

Colorectal cancer can derive from causes similar to those of constipation, but with a more critical and more in-depth emotional factor. In the case of constipation, it is the most superficial energies or emotions that intervene. Still, in the case of cancer, the cause must be sought in the strengths and passions located in the deepest part of our being.

WHAT DO I DO?

If you suspect you may have colorectal cancer, the first step is to "go to the doctor." This is by far the most crucial step for us or for anyone who may have this disease.

Going to the doctor quickly and responsibly is the best option to establish an accurate diagnosis and initiate adequate and timely treatment, but: Where do I go?

"Where to go" is, perhaps, what worries us most and, without a doubt, one of the most critical factors for your recovery. Knowing who can help or guide in this decision is both a cause of high anxiety and anguish.

In most cases, in the presence of signs and symptoms such as bleeding or anal pain, you should go quickly to our first option, usually our family or trusted doctor. This often represents an internist, gastroenterologist, or general surgeon, but are they the best option to guide me and/or help me?

The answer is "YES," our trusted doctors will always be helpful and can give us excellent recommendations. However, we must ask ourselves if there is another group of doctors who specializes in diseases of the colon, rectum, and anus.

Yes, they exist. At this time, colorectal surgeons are specialized in the management of diseases of the colon, rectum, and anus. Therefore, they can be chosen to treat patients with colorectal cancer. The most important thing is: stay with that doctor (Colorectal surgeons, gastroenterologist, or oncologist surgeon) that generates TRUST. Someone who, with their attention, makes us feel safe and peaceful, gives us hope, understands us, and is willing to accompany us. Because at the end of this story, the only thing I can choose is who to trust or in a more profound way: to whom can I say, "You are my doctor!"

There are many treatment protocols for colorectal cancer and deciding which one is best for our particular case is the task of the medical team that we choose. They will pick it and will guide us through the treatment option to be proposed. We simply must find an excellent medical team that transmits security and confidence. We can consider options; we can listen to advise from our family and friends. But, once again, the only real choice is to decide with which medical team I want to treat my illness, the rest is simply a matter of faith because I must trust that they will do their best.

WHERE DO I FIND IT?

The key to choose our treating medical team would be to look for those assistance centers or specialized units with a high volume of patients and with experience. Experience and constant practice have an essential role since in these centers, large multidisciplinary work teams are composed of coloproctologists, oncologists, radiotherapists, pathologists, gastroenterologists, general surgeons, laparoscopists, internists, cardiologists, nutritionists, psychologists, among others.

The integration of these specialties offer comprehensive and quality care in these centers. This combination is what provides optimal treatment and will help us overcome the disease.

It is proven that better results are obtained in patient survival and lower morbidity and mortality rates when diagnosis and therapy are implemented in specialized medical centers with high patient volume, and that includes multidisciplinary medical groups.

WHO COMES WITH ME?

This is a vital, disturbing question, cuz it can be hard for many people to choose a family member or friend with whom to go to the doctor. It is a simple task, but not all of us have excellent family support. And not all of our relatives have the empathy to help us to face this type of situation.

Given the suspicion of disease as multifactorial as cancer, the most important thing is not to go to the doctor's office alone. However, the best company must be a person we trust and who, also, can provide us with unconditional support and help us to understand the indications given by the doctor clearly. Someone who can help us clarify the information with the doctor because we might feel bewildered by this hard news.

The indicated person must have the necessary emotional maturity to ask the pertinent questions to the doctor and be able to transmit the information in the best possible way. Above all, it must be someone who helps us carry the burden, that gives us hope, that allows us to understand the situation we are in.

HOW DO I DECIDE WHERE TO GO?

The most important thing is to make the decision to go to the doctor. Although repetitive, that decision can be challenging to make, and yet this gives us a more significant opportunity to establish the diagnosis in time or rule out other diseases.

It is important to remember that our trusted doctor is in the ability to guide us about the condition and can also recommend "where to go."

When it comes to colorectal cancer, it is best to go with a "colorectal surgeon" or "coloproctologist" since they are the ones specialized in the treatment of diseases of the colon, rectum, and anus. They can perform and analyze all relevant studies to establish the precise diagnosis and also guide us step by step in all the stages of the process that involve the treatment of this disease, from the contact with the multidisciplinary team for the studies of pathological anatomy, psychological support for our relatives and us, the indication of administration of chemotherapy and radiotherapy, until the definitive surgical intervention in case of meriting it.

WHAT NOT TO DO?

If we were to write a list of the 15 things that should not be done in the presence of signs and symptoms suggestive of colorectal cancer, the first 10 recommendations would inevitably say something like: "I should NOT keep quiet in the presence of symptoms" and the following 5 something like: "I must not wait to go to the doctor" and finally they would be phrases opposite to "IF I HAVE PAIN OR RECTAL BLEEDING I SHOULD COME QUICKLY TO THE DOCTOR AND TELL HIM WHAT I FEEL."

Early consultation without hesitation gives us the "best opportunity" to know whether or not we have cancer and the best therapeutic option to cure us.

WHAT CAN I FEEL?

For all of us, there must be multiple answers, feelings, and significant uncertainties about it. We are sure that the first thing is that we will feel "fear," fear of pain, fear of suffering, fear of loneliness, fear of losing our loved ones, fear of death. The important thing would be to know how can I feel?

The signs and symptoms that occur due to colorectal cancer are nonspecific, often accompanied by changes in the evacuation habit and stool shape. What does this mean?

It means that we should suspect a possible colorectal cancer if we notice any change in the frequency of our bowel movements. If we present with constipation or diarrhea without apparent causes, alterations in the form of feces, which, in most cases, they can become fragmented and small or thin, similar to "tapes."

Also, anal or anorectal pain and bleeding before, during, and even after bowel movements, can be signs that raise alarms to suspect malignant disease in the colon or rectum. We must be careful because many ignore the initial manifestations of the disease, which is a delay factor for the diagnosis.

In this context, the observations we make as patients are more important than any medical interrogation.

WHAT COULD BE, AND WHAT NOT?

Many times we feel that things happen to others cannot affect us, or otherwise, everything that happens to others, is something I also suffer. Both extremes of thinking can become harmful. The final idea is that If I feel a mass in the anorectum or I have bleeding or pain when having a bowel movement or even a sensation of anorectal weight, tenesmus or difficulty in expelling stool, I should not panic or be out of control and completely alarmed because I have cancer. Still, I'm not going to be home carefree because "my neighbor says they are hemorrhoids."

The truth is that of many pathologies that affect the colon, rectum, and anus —such as hemorrhoids, anal fissures, abscesses, and anorectal fistulas, diverticular disease, angiodysplasia, among others— that are benign in nature. However, a large percentage of patients who experience a sensation of palpable masses, pain, bleeding, and changes in the consistency/shape of stool and the evacuation pattern are diagnosed with colon or rectal cancer, especially in elderly patients.

CHAPTER II:

❋ ❋ ❋

How to know?

DO I WANNA KNOW?

Many of us when we go to the doctor direct our expectations to know "if we can be cured or not" without knowing when we have to ask "Doctor, I understand that I have cancer, but can I be cured?". And this is not an easy question to ask.

The answer to this question goes beyond its simple formulation because it is clear that I need to feel safe and raise my hopes.

It is necessary to know that something can be done with this disease, that we can be cured, that it is not terminal, that we can continue to enjoy our lives and share it with our loved ones. Still, to achieve all this, it is necessary to overcome fear and, the only way to do it is: "Learning to know my cancer."

As patients, you can be of great help to your doctors, and you have the most considerable authority to tell them about your evolution during the disease. Still, to be able to help you, you need to know about what you have. It is necessary to understand what cancer is.

Cancer is a generic term used to describe a broad group of diseases that can affect any part of the body. There are also known synonymous as "malignant tumors" or "malignant neoplasms."

A peculiar characteristic of cancer is the fast multiplication of abnormal cells capable of extending beyond their region of origin and can invade adjacent parts or spread to other organs. This is a process known as "metastasis," these metastases being the leading cause of death. Now, do I really want or, do I need to know all this information?

The answer to the previous question is "YES," a resounding and gigantic "YES!".

Any of us feels immense fear for the thought of getting cancer. The vast majority of us "block" this possibility, and we think there's "no way out" when they give us this hard news.

This is innate to the human being. We are terrified of what we do not know, and, generally, we make the mistake of falling into "denial." Refusing to accept what is happening in our bodies, conditions us physically, mentally, and spiritually to make bad decisions in our lives.

When we make the decision to go to a doctor, it is because we already know that something is wrong. We probably already suspect that something is happening, but behind the fear, uncertainty, and denial, the truth is hidden.

Denying that I have cancer is the easiest way I can escape from reality. To believe that this can happen to others and not to me, to think that the doctor was wrong and that I should seek help elsewhere. Maybe at another time, maybe when I feel better, but everything takes me away from the possibility of timely treatment that can give me complete healing.

Understanding and accepting is not easy, but it is important to know what is happening in our body will open the way to healing. We must know what we are facing, "I want to know why I want to heal!"

As doctors, we shall tell that, on many occasions, we shared with patients that when they are told their diagnosis, they do not record in their thinking what they are told. It seems that they are disconnected, blocked, do not want to know, they should not know and less understand. It looks a little like the effect that is generated when a human body receives a significant physical impact: the pain is immense, and later a pious anesthetic effect occurs, and pain is not felt.

It is a fact that cancer does not disappear by magic, does not go away, and then returns years later. It does not appear, it grows and then lives in communion with our bodies. Cancer stays, grows, destroys tissues and organs, and the best way to deal with it is by taking responsibility for myself that I have cancer. I cannot deny my reality. I cannot block myself from receiving help, looking for alternatives, and taking the recommendations that my doctor has to help me.

WHAT IF I DON'T
WANT TO KNOW?

Many times we are entirely sure that ignoring the truth is better for us, but there is no more wrong and dangerous thought than this. It is possible that many times we feel blocked, scared, depressed, and end up rejecting that reality so distressing that having cancer is. In these moments, we must ask ourselves, do I really not want to know what I have?, am I merely rejecting my illness?, or am I afraid of death?

Most human beings are not prepared to receive difficult news, news that we do not want to hear or are not trained to handle. If this is your case, we want to tell you something beautiful: "you are not alone." Blocking and hiding in the face of adversity is a common denominator for many. Still, the important thing here is to understand that we are not alone.

Denying the reality we face will only have negative consequences: delays in diagnosis, delays in treatment, in medical care. Refusing will only take our loved ones and us away from the right steps to follow. We lose the invaluable resource of time and will not focus our energies on our healing.

Our family, friends, doctors, therapists, psychologists, and, to a large extent, our spiritual beliefs can help us take a step towards acceptance.

So what if we change this paradigm? And, instead of asking ourselves "what if I don't want to know?", we say we are sure of ourselves, "I want to know!", "I need to know!" "I have to act!".

WHERE IS IT, AND HOW IS IT?

Come on! If we are ready to know, there will be many doubts at the beginning. Where is it? What is it? How did it happen? Can I wait? What studies should I be undergoing?

Where is it? It is one of the most disturbing questions. Especially since we must know that depending on the segment of the intestine where the tumor is found, the treatment schemes for our healing may vary.

Most types of cancer in the human body receive their name from the organ where they originate. In this case, colorectal cancer has this name because it originates in the last portion of the digestive tract that is made up of the colon and rectum.

The colon begins where the small intestine ends. Its primary function is the absorption of water from ingested food and the production of fecal matter with the help of its own bacterial flora: an essential set of bacteria that live in harmony and naturally with the colon and help it to perform many of his vital functions.

The colon is divided into five segments whose names are: cecum (where the cecal appendix is found), ascending colon, hepatic angle, transverse colon, splenic angle, descending colon and sigmoid colon, is approximately 120 cm long in most people, and the rectal (rectum), a blister that measures another 15 cm is continued.

Likewise, these different portions of the colon can be divided into two large sets with the midline of the body and thus grouped into a "right colon" (cecum, ascending and the right half of the transverse) and a "left colon" (half left of transverse, descending and sigmoid)

The rectum is the last portion of the large intestine, and its primary function is to serve as a reservoir to store stool before its evacuation. It begins as a continuation of the sigmoid colon and ends after joining the anal canal in the anorectal junction.

The rectum can be divided into three anatomical portions, upper, medium, and low. However, for practical purposes of its study and treatment, they are commonly recognized as an upper rectum and a low rectum.

Approximately 20% of colon cancers develop in the cecum, 25% in the sigmoid colon, 20% for rectum, and an additional 10% in the junction of the sigmoid colon with the rectum, or also known as the rectosigmoid junction.

Both the colon and the rectum are formed by a circular wall composed of multiple layers of different tissues. We are going to illustrate it quickly: if we cut a plastic tube transversely, we could have an example of what the colon and rectum wall looks like with a hollow center and solid structures on the walls.

These layers, from the inside out, are called: mucosa, submucosa, muscular and serous layer, each of them with fundamental characteristics and properties for the proper functioning of the organ. Cancer originates in the innermost layer, that is, the mucosa, and can grow through each of these layers until it extends well beyond the colon and rectum and invades other body structures.

Knowing about these layers is of vital importance since the severity, stage, or extent of colorectal cancer depends on the number of layers that are affected by the tumor. Thanks to this, your doctor can know how advanced is the disease, and this may help to establish a stage diagnosis.

WHAT DOES IT MEAN "STAGES" OF COLORECTAL CANCER?

Stage diagnosis is the process by which the doctor, through individual studies, establishes the degree of disease progression at the time of diagnosis. This helps to choose the strategy and sequence of treatment that suits our situation. To do so, the number of layers that are taken or "infiltrated," the lymph node involvement and the presence of distant disease or "metastasis" is taken into account.

Simply put, classification by stages is the most accurate way to establish how far cancer has spread in our body. This is extremely important since the chances of successful treatment and total healing have a relationship with the stage you are in.

Likewise, establishing the stage at the time of diagnosis helps us evaluate our long-term life expectancy. This has been determined through numerous studies in cancer patients who build, through reliable statistics, the percentage of patients who remain healthy and/or alive in the first 5 years after diagnosis and treatment.

Systems classify the stages of colorectal cancer using a series of numbers and letters to establish each grade. These determine the spread of the disease through the layers that make up the wall of the organ, as well as the invasion of other neighboring areas or structures.

The stages are identified with Roman numerals from I to IV (1 to 4). In turn, each number is subdivided into several groups, identified with letters that generally go from A to C.

In the particular case of colorectal cancer, numbers I and II apply to those tumors that do not invade lymph nodes, number III for those involving the nodes, and IV for metastatic or distant disease. The letters are used within each group of numbers to make the invasion and compromise of the different tissues and/or structures involved more specific.

An accurate initial staging can influence the treatment by helping to determine the type of surgical intervention and the choice of neoadjuvant therapy. That is, the initial chemotherapy or radiotherapy scheme, if necessary, to maximize the possibility of healing and survival for each patient.

For early-stage malignant tumors, surgery may be all that is needed to solve the problem. For more advanced cancers, other treatments, such as chemotherapy or radiotherapy, could be added. However, for most patients, the definitive stage is not determined precisely until after the surgical resection of the tumor, so the doctor could wait until after surgery to inform us about the final stage.

We should not hesitate to ask our doctor about the stage in which the disease is, the options or combinations of treatment available, and how can we achieve the best results and ensure our cure.

ARE THERE DIFFERENT TYPES OF COLORECTAL CANCER?

The answer to this question is YES, it depends on the cells and tissues determined by the histological study. There are different types of malignant tumors in the colon and rectum, depending on the tissue where the tumor cells originally formed. This is done by the Pathologist, a specialist responsible for determining the origin of various diseases through the study of affected tissues.

Cancer that is generated in different segments of the colon or rectum can cause different symptoms and affect us in various ways.

Colorectal cancer usually originates from premalignant lesions such as polyps. A polyp is a mass of abnormal, but typically benign, tissue that grows slowly (over several years), originating in the mucous layer of the intestine.

Polyps are also known as adenomas and can occur in different sizes, shapes and types. Some with a higher degree of malignancy than others. Early removal of the polyp is the best way to prevent its progression to cancer, hence the importance of conducting endoscopic studies when indicated.

The vast majority (98%) of malignant tumors in the colon and rectum are adenocarcinomas (ADC). The remaining (2%), rare varieties such as lymphomas (1.3%), carcinoid tumors (0.4%), and sarcomas (0.3%), each of these has different behaviors, treatments, and responses. The ADC is the most common, and it has an excellent response to treatment and better survival, especially if it is diagnosed and treated in the earliest stages of the disease.

HOW IS COLORECTAL CANCER DIAGNOSED?

To doctors, it is vital what we, as patients, can provide when referring to what we feel or care about. It is, —the patients— we who give our doctors the first clues that they need to make the diagnosis of the disease.

Experts say that a careful evaluation before the establishment of the diagnosis or treatment of patients with colorectal cancer is essential for the successful management of the disease, but:

HOW CAN THE DOCTOR DIAGNOSE THIS DISEASE?

The initial evaluation for the diagnosis begins like any medical evaluation: with a good conversation! Where we will tell the doctor everything we feel and live so that he can make an excellent clinical history of our disease.

The interview, conversation, and interactions we have with our doctor are fundamental elements for a proper doctor-patient relationship. This newly formed team will go through hard, stressful periods, impregnated with obstacles, pains, and loss of faith. Still, they are also necessary for bonding and allowing interrelation, understanding, and cooperation in the sequences of a diagnostic and therapeutic process that may last many years.

The next step is also simple; it consists of a complete physical examination and, although it may seem uncomfortable. An adequate coloproctological examination consists of a rectal examination and anoscopy. Anoscopy consists of introducing an instrument similar to a speculum into the anal canal to be able to evaluate the structures of the anal canal and lower rectum. Additionally, a rectoscopy may be performed to observe a little higher in the rectal ampulla.

The coloproctologist has enough experience and delicacy to

minimize the discomfort we may feel. We should not worry about feeling pain or discomfort during the physical examination in the anorectal region.

Also, it is necessary to perform a gynecological exam in women. This is done in a complementary, simple way at the doctor's office without special preparation unless the proctologist indicates otherwise. Do not worry, the evaluation can be straightforward and accurate in expert hands with a minimum of discomfort or pain.

Once our medical record is created, and all crucial data have been established, it is necessary to rely on technology to help complete our evaluation. For this, numerous resources will help the doctor to know more fully what we can have, we just have to be precise. What are these resources? What studies can my doctor do to help me?

The most commonly used study to evaluate colorectal cancer are colonoscopy and tomography. In the particular case of rectal cancer, 3D endorectal ultrasound and magnetic resonance imaging can be performed. Likewise, laboratory tests to evaluate our general condition and the determination of tumor markers such as the carcinoembryonic antigen (CEA).

ENDOSCOPIC STUDIES

Colonoscopy is a study through which an endoscope (tube with a camera) is inserted through the rectum to inspect the entire large intestine in real-time. It is the safest method to detect early colorectal cancer because it allows you to explore the intestinal mucosa in detail and assess its status.

It also offers the possibility of taking biopsies in those segments of the mucosa that are suspected of tumors. Additionally, it allows the removal of possible polyps that could be found and taking all these tissue "biopsies" or "samples" for study and diagnosis in pathology.

Colonoscopy is indicated in every person over 50 years of age regardless of whether they have risk factors or not and, in all those over 35 years who have associated risk factors for colorectal cancer.

An important aspect when we talk about any study, especially the endoscopic ones, is to know if we must perform or undergo a previous preparation. In this case, to make a colonoscopy, the colon must be perfectly clean by proper training before the procedure.

How is this preparation done?

Is it tough to get a colon preparation? Will I feel pain?

Preparing for a colonoscopy is not difficult or painful, perhaps a bit annoying or uncomfortable, especially since we will have to evacuate many times. Still, it is something that will not last more than 24 hours.

The day before the study you should not eat foods that are difficult to digest or that cause gas but maintain a diet with clear liquids and leave no thew will not be residues in the colon. If the exploration is carried out in the morning (preferably), we must begin the evacuation of the bowel from 2:00 p.m. on the previous day. From that moment, we should have a liquid diet consisting mainly of tea, water, or clear soups. Coffee, juices, and dairy products are not allowed. The night before the colonoscopy, you should not have dinner.

The preparation includes taking two to four liters of laxative solution in a 90-minute interval starting the previous afternoon. The morning of the study, an evacuation enema is applied until the evacuations consist of a transparent liquid with no residue.

It is necessary to completely empty the intestine because, otherwise, the state of the mucosa in the intestine wall won't be fully assessed, which is the objective of the study.

The bowel movement procedure is perceived as a stressful process, and, in fact, it is so. It is a bit annoying to go to the bathroom continually. At the same time, the intestine empties remember that it is something necessary and completely harmless that will only last a few hours so, we have nothing to worry about!

The colonoscopy lasts between 15 and 45 minutes. In most cases, we are given a sedative and, if necessary, an analgesic.

After the exploration, you can immediately eat again what pleases you! But you should not do activities that require high concentration, like driving directly after the procedure due to the effects of sedation and some likely discomfort. Therefore, it is best to go accompanied by a family member or a good friend to take you back home.

IMAGE STUDIES

The most essential imaging study is currently the tomography of the abdomen and pelvis with double contrast, that is, using a contrast medium ingested orally, and another injected intravenously. This study allows the exploration of the entire abdominal and pelvic cavity through the use of tomography. This will take multiple images with millimeter cuts of the whole area to be evaluated through x-rays. This will let us know how our body is internally.

The tomography does not require prior preparation of the colon. It is necessary to maintain a liquid diet the day before the study and ingest the contrast medium by mouth at least 4 to 12 hours before the examination. It is possible that the contrast has a strange taste and causes some nausea. Still, the few discomforts that can be generated are temporary and do not merit any treatment in most cases.

You might get an abdominal ultrasound (US) before tomography. It is a faster study and can be done directly in the office, to know if our solid intra-abdominal organs, especially the liver, have alterations like a metastasis. Still, tomography is the most suitable study for this purpose.

Surely many of us are familiar with ultrasound because it is a routine procedure for many conditions such as evaluation during pregnancy, but there are currently special devices for the ultrasound evaluation of specific organs such as 3D endorectal ultrasound (US ER3D) which in some cancers —particularly rectum—, it is necessary

This is an ultrasonographic study where a device (transducer) is introduced through the anal canal, evaluating the layers of the rectum and its relationship with neighboring structures.

It is an innocuous procedure and quite well tolerated by the majority of patients, perhaps a little uncomfortable due to the fact of introducing an object into the rectum, but with a short duration.

The US ER3D is a handy tool to know the involvement or infiltration that the tumor has on the walls of the rectum. It allows evaluating ganglia presence and penetration to adjacent structures such as the wall of the vagina or the prostate.

The preparation for the endorectal ultrasound only requires the application of an evacuation enema 2-4 hours before the test. It is not necessary to go on an empty stomach, we can eat normally, and it is not required to go with any companion. Endorectal ultrasound has no known risks or contraindications. We can continue our daily activities immediately after exploration.

Finally, we can use the MRI resource that, like the US 3D, is used for the staging of rectal cancer. Both procedures have a comparable utility between them; therefore, resonance is only indicated in particular conditions, primarily to assess the anatomy of the entire pelvis more accurately.

LABORATORY EXAMS

The usefulness of blood lab tests really is quite straightforward. Complete hematology, glycemia, urea, creatinine, serum electrolytes, cholesterol levels, triglycerides, bilirubin, transaminases, among many others, are useful to know the general clinical conditions of each patient. Still, the most valuable for us is the determination of the CEA.

The carcinoembryonic antigen, or CEA, is a tumor marker that rises mainly in the presence of malignant pathologies in the colon and rectum and is a prognostic marker of treatment response, cure or recurrence (appearance of new cancer cells). Its average value is <5 IU in non-smoking patients and <10 IU in smokers.

Current guidelines recommend that all patients with colorectal cancer should be evaluated with a CT scan, complete colonoscopy, and carcinoembryonic antigen, as well as US ER3D or MRI of the pelvis in the specific context of rectal cancer.

Other studies to be considered are chest radiography or chest tomography, if necessary, and positron emission tomography (CT-PET). The latter is reserved for patients with specific conditions during the evaluation, except for the Chest x-ray that is done routinely.

CHAPTER III:

How is it treated?

Accurate diagnosis allows you to be prepared for a decision. It is crucial to keep in mind that our doctor will explain the treatment options according to what can generate better results. We, as patients, must do everything possible to adapt and accept the treatments indicated because the objective of all this is: beat cancer!

Many treatment alternatives are available today. However, we must remember that each patient is different, and some therapies are better suited to some than others.

Already at this stage, we will begin to hear words such as surgery, chemotherapy, radiotherapy, colostomy, margins, resection, even terms such as adjuvant, neoadjuvant, survival, complications, and others that will surely confuse us. But this is the most appropriate time to know and understand the things that can happen.

CAN I BE CURED?

This is, without a doubt, the most crucial question for you, for your family members, for your life. The one that, without fear of mistakes, causes more uncertainty, worry, and anxiety than any other that any of us can think of. So, we have a convenient answer and that, when you decide to believe it, will radically change our way of appreciating life. Then you wonder if you can beat cancer and the good news is that the answer is: YES!

We can cure ourselves, we can get ahead and defeat cancer! There are many alternatives, from some long and complicated roads to simple solutions with minimal changes in our lifestyle.

However, to overcome "cancer," it is crucial to specify the staging at the time of diagnosis, knowing where it is and how the injury will allow us to plan the strategy to succeed!

Nine out of ten people, who are detected and treated early colorectal cancer, can be cured entirely and without significant consequences. Hence the importance of establishing an early diagnosis of the disease.

On the other hand, if cancer has spread to the lymph nodes or to other organs, healing and survival could be affected. However, it is necessary to emphasize that there is always a treatment option. There will always be possibilities to continue enjoying the blessing of sharing the world with our loved ones.

Although survival rates are generally calculated at 5 years, these statistics vary for each patient. We must take into account that each person is unique and statistics only give us a general idea of how a disease can develop. The vast majority of patients with colorectal cancer live for more than 5 years, especially if the diagnosis is established early. So we must remember: statistics cannot predict what will happen in each case!

When in doubt or questions about our chances of healing, we need to ask ourselves: Do I really want to be guided by statistics or, do I want to have the courage to go further and fight (with all my faith and strength) to heal? After answering this, we can go to our medical team and tell them: I have the conviction that I will heal myself and my healing possibilities are endless! Let's work together!

Be sure that our family members, our doctors, and friends, admiring our determination and courage, will feel admiration and love. This will generate the energy needed to continue moving forward.

WHAT DO I DO FIRST?

How to explain in a few words the steps to follow or, what action should we take first? This is a complicated thing to define, but we could use five words to accomplish this task successfully: think, decide, act, believe, and trust.

The important thing is to select our medical team. It is time to make a decision. We must take into account the results of studies carried out, analyze the advantages and what each procedure means according to our expectations, consider the experience of the treating medical team at each step of the treatment and listen to the opinion of our family.

We must know that depending on the tumor location, the treatment that can be offered will be unique; different portions of the colon and rectum will have surgical and oncological strategies that best fit each of them, with better survival and fewer complications than others.

The job of the medical and surgical team is to offer the best treatment options for our healing and well-being!

Whether we have to undergo an initial surgical treatment or receive prior treatment with chemotherapy or radiotherapy, we must trust that the treatment chosen by our doctors is appropriate. This certainty will give us the courage and energy to obtain the best results.

The results are linked to your faith in your ability to win.

CAN I BE HEALED?

To heal, we must begin to do it from within, from the deepest part of our being. Heal ourselves. We must first understand that healing depends only on us and on our positive and successful attitude towards illness.

This is how we can say that to start our healing process, the first step is to accept our disease. This is essential to undertake the "fight" against cancer. The proposal is to understand and ask myself the question: If I refuse to accept my illness, how can I work on my healing?

Understanding our diagnosis, accepting it, and deciding to overcome it are vital steps to success!

I accept to drop old attitudes and change my perception of life, understand that I am valuable to myself and others, open my heart, and become aware of all that life can give me.

We can share with family and friends, receive a massage, eat what we like, read books, listen to our favorite music or, any other distraction that makes us feel at ease. It will have the effect of such an intoxicating harmonization that will allow us to open our consciences to all the wonders of life and beauties that surround us. This will strengthen us physically and mentally and will take us to a higher level, from our spiritual energy to our immune system.

WILL I HAVE SURGERY?

Surgery is almost always an unavoidable treatment in the case of colorectal cancer if we ask ourselves the initial question of whether or not to have surgery. Still, a surgeon might answer: it depends. But this term "depends" is not a sign of insecurity; it is instead a sign of maturity and wisdom on their part.

Let's expand this concept:

There are several types of treatment for colorectal cancer: surgery, radiotherapy, chemotherapy, immunotherapy, and even others depending on the stage of the disease. Surgery is used as an initial and only treatment, another option is a combination of chemotherapy plus radiation therapy without surgery or a combination of all.

Surgery has the function of eliminating the most considerable amount of tumor mass from our body. For this purpose, surgical options vary from local resection (removing the tumor from the internal surface of the colon or rectum) to extended resection of the tumor including, other organs close to this portion of the digestive tract.

On the other hand, chemotherapy and radiotherapy can be applied before surgery in some cases, and this is what is called neo-adjuvant. Its function is to decrease tumor size and its extension to other neighboring organs, allowing the surgeon for a better resection being able to preserve more disease-free tissue.

Even some patients with low rectal cancer may respond so dramatically to the combined treatment of chemotherapy and neoadjuvant radiotherapy that after reassessing their response they won't need surgery. Still, they must remain under medical control and surveillance for some time. They would avoid being subjected to the surgical procedure.

IS IT OPERABLE?
WHERE, HOW,
AND WHEN?

The decision is based on tumor location and disease conditions in each particular patient at the time of diagnosis. The objective is to achieve the best balance between the quality of life and the appropriate treatments. The aim is to restore bowel and evacuation function as similar to normal.

Despite how complex it might be to answer the question: How are the colon and rectum operated? We could come to understand in general what these procedures are and how they differ from each other. We propose that you accept that colon and rectum are two different structures for the surgical resection extension.

HOW IS COLON OPERATED?

After determining the extent of the disease, we can divide it into several forms of presentation taking into account the place where it is and how it affects the intestine itself and its relationship with adjacent organs:

1- Resectable And Non-Obstructive Tumors.

This is perhaps the least complicated form of the disease. These are all tumors that have not spread to other neighboring or distant organs. It can be safely removed surgically since it has not yet caused an acute intestinal obstruction. Intestinal obstruction is defined as the inability to pass stool from one to another intestinal segment due to a blockage by a tumor.

In these cases, it's recommended to perform a complete resection of the segment of the colon compromised with its corresponding arteries, veins, and lymphatic vessels. This is what is known in medical language as: "radical surgery."

If a tumor is on the right or left portion of the colon, it can be resected whole in the form of a hemicolectomy (right hemicolectomy or left hemicolectomy), that is, removing half of the colon where the tumor is located. Then the ends of the sectioned intestine can be joined to maintain the continuity of the digestive tract; this union is called "anastomosis."

In the particular case of the sigmoid colon, it can be radically resected on its own, and anastomosis of the colon to the rectum is performed.

Sometimes it is not possible to perform the binding of the remaining bowel segments, and the anastomosis is postponed for a second surgery. In these cases, an ostomy is performed, which consists of exteriorizing a part of the intestine through the abdominal wall, where evacuations will be passed temporarily or permanently.

The possibility of an ostomy is something that we should talk extensively with our medical team before surgery. You should plan its location and understand how we should handle it. We will discuss ostomies in more detail later.

2 - Resectable But Tumor Complicated With Intestinal Obstruction:

These are all those tumors in which the growth towards the intestinal lumen occludes (obstructs) the passage of feces and produces the absence of bowel movements. This is accompanied by abdominal pain and vomiting, which can last several days of evolution and represent a surgical emergency.

Perhaps this complication is one of the most worrisome for our loved ones and us. Because we always hear rumors or know some history that someone was in bad condition or died due to intestinal obstruction. In many cases, this could be a complication, but we must bear in mind that this occurs because patients refrain to go to the doctor for a long time after it happens.

Therefore, if a possible intestinal obstruction is suspected and in the case of a diagnosis of colorectal cancer, we should promptly turn to our medical team.

On the other hand, in some cases, intestinal obstruction is the first sign and/or symptom that occurs when you have colon or rectal cancer. This is mainly because these tumors have slow growth and are not visible to the naked eye, which contributes to the fact that the diagnosis is not always made early. Even sometimes, the diagnosis is established after intestinal obstruction surgery from an unknown cause.

The importance of this is that having an emergency is a challenge for the surgical team, increasing the likelihood of performing ostomies. However, the medical team will explain in detail the risks of emergency surgery, as well as the necessary steps to prepare the intervention. The surgeon and his medical team can make several decisions during the surgery: 1- resect the tumor radically and perform the anastomosis. 2- resect the tumor radically and perform an ostomy. 3- place a stent, that is, a prosthesis can be inserted into the lumen of the intestine to allow the passage of feces temporarily until surgical resolution is possible. The diversity of decisions depends on the conditions in which the emergency arises and on our general clinical conditions.

3 - Tumor With Metastasis.

These are tumors that have been in our body for a long time and have spread to other structures invading the liver, lungs, and brain more frequently.

In these cases, the medical team most likely recommends receiving treatment before performing any surgery.

There are drug schemes that reduce the number of tumor cells present in the colon and the organs to which they have spread. The administration of these "chemotherapy" schemes before surgery is called "neoadjuvant chemotherapy." The evaluation of their effect by the medical team will allow, if possible, to subsequently perform a radical surgery with a higher probability of cure. Also, they will improve symptoms related to tumor invasion.

4 - Unresectable Tumor.

These are all those with invasion to adjacent structures, like other portions of the digestive system or important vascular structures that make resection impossible without compromising the life of the patients.

5 - Inoperable Tumor.

Those patients in whom, regardless of tumor extension or infiltration, can not be taken to surgical intervention due to aggravating medical conditions.

HOW IS THE RECTUM OPERATED?

There are different treatment alternatives for the colon and rectum.

It is necessary to remember that tumors in the rectum can be "high" or "low" depending on the anatomical location they have in this organ.

Tumors located in the upper rectum, that is, those that are not reachable by the doctor's digital touch can be treated in the same way as colon lesions are treated. In contrast, tumors that are in the lower rectum or, slightly, those that are less than 8cm from the margin of the anus and that can be touched by rectal examination will have different treatment schedules.

1- Low Rectal Tumors Complicated With Intestinal Obstruction.

These can be considered an emergency and often have a relatively high percentage of infiltration to adjacent tissues and organs. Some can receive treatment before surgery (neoadjuvant), with chemotherapy and radiotherapy.

Intestinal obstruction is usually treated with the creation of a temporary ostomy to evacuate while receiving neoadjuvant treatment.

2 - Small Tumors Near The Anal Margin And With Little Infiltration To The Tissues.

These may be resected with relative "greater ease" through the anus, without compromising the principle of radicality in cancer surgery. This procedure is known as: "transanal local excision" and recovery period is quicker.

Generally, tumors with an indication of this resection are diagnosed early and in early disease stages.

Likewise, these tumors can also be operated through the abdomen, resecting the entire diseased rectum and rejoining the colon to the remaining portion through an anastomosis. Generally, the anastomosis is performed between the descending colon and the anal canal passing through the anorectal sphincter apparatus. The anal sphincters are muscles that allow to maintain the continence of the feces and prevent them from coming out by themselves. this will keep the evacuation in a physiological form, and this procedure is known as "sphincter-preserving surgery."

In the particular case of rectal tumors, there are special considerations that translate into good news for us. Many times the tumors have such an excellent response to treatment with chemotherapy and radiotherapy that they reduce and disappear entirely from our body and do not require surgery. This is known as a "complete tumor response."

However, as stated above, patients who are lucky enough to get this response must undergo strict medical control for at least 5 years, and, if all goes well, they won't be requiring surgery at any time. What would happen if the tumor does not respond to neoadjuvant therapy? What happens if the response to treatment is not complete? What happens if cancer grows again? What happens if a tumor is too low, or too close to the anal margin and compromises the sphincter apparatus?

In these cases, surgical treatment is our only option. Still, without discouragement ! even if it is the "only option," the essential thing is that there is always an option! The detail here would be: What kind of surgical procedure could I have?

For this, our surgeon will resort to a procedure created years ago at the beginning of the 20th century. Nevertheless, we should not worry. Despite being a somewhat "old" technique, this has evolved since its origins, and, at this time, it is safe and reliable surgery.

The problem that we could find is that the abdominal-perineal resection, as this technique is known, involves the resection of the rectal tumor by the abdominal route and also by the perineal way. The perineum is the lower region or floor of our pelvis, it is the area where we can see the anus. Therefore, we could never evacuate through the anus again, and we would have a definitive colostomy. This is a small thing considering how little it is to have a colostomy for life if we can continue to live many more years!

WHAT HAPPENS IF, AFTER SURGERY, THERE ARE TRACES OF THE TUMOR IN OUR BODY?

If this happens, the first thing we should do is: don't be alarmed!

We must remain calm and our mind positive, continue to believe faithfully in our complete, absolute, and definitive healing.

However sometimes, especially in situations where the tumor resection margins are narrow, it may happen that tumor resection margins are not wide enough or are "compromised." It means there is the presence of tumor at the cutting edge, so tumor particles may remain in the healthy intestine. For this situation, there are the postoperative or "adjuvant" treatment schemes that will accomplish the elimination of the tumor cells that were left in our body.

Adjuvant therapy is indicated when there are infiltrated lymph nodes in the result of a definitive biopsy report or by molecular characteristics of tumors. This does not mean that it is a bad thing for us, but we must use this tool to ensure adequate and definitive treatment.

WHAT TO DO IF THE DISEASE IS VERY ADVANCED? WHEN IS IT TOO LATE FOR US?

We firmly believe that we should begin this section by stating that: IT IS NEVER TOO LATE!

Sometimes we hear words so hopeless and unpleasant about our medical condition that, even with all the strength and faith we have, we feel that the world is upon us. We must be alert because these words often come from our own doctor or our loved ones. However, we have to understand that it's never too late to keep fighting!

Patients who present inoperable or unresectable tumors, with distant or advanced disease, should consider that there are always alternatives. It is not the end of the world. The important thing is not to give up and focus our energy on seeking to heal our body and soul. All that matters is enjoying our lives and the company of our loved ones in complete freedom and harmony.

Although cancer in advanced stages represents an extraordinary challenge for the treating medical team, there are always treatment protocols that can be applied to patients with this degree of commitment. The goal of chemotherapy or radiotherapy treatments is the possibility of turning an inoperable patient into an operable one. Or, at least, allowing them to enjoy a better quality of life.

CHAPTER IV:

* * *

What's going to happen?

K nowing what can happen to each of us is difficult to predict. However, the most important thing is to know that we can do something to win that hard battle against cancer.

Imagining what we can feel or the experiences that we are going to live is something that will depend only on us and on the attitude with which we face this problem. Cancer is not an easy disease to overcome, but it is one that can be overcome!

The way we face the problems in our lives is vital to find a quick and satisfactory solution. Hence, a positive and fighting attitude is an excellent tool to rise above any obstacle.

Even though our attitude is the best, and even if we are the bravest and most determined, we can not ignore the concern and uncertainty for not knowing what awaits us on the road. We may be terrified to our bone for not knowing: What will I feel? What can we feel during this stage? What can we do to feel better?

The best way to know what we could feel is to try to talk with people who have been through the same as us, seek help, read a book, research on the internet, read an article.

Many publications talk about the stages of cancer and how to deal with them and live with them. Still, we could say that the best way to deal with cancer is with faith and hope, faith in God, in our families, friends, doctors, ourselves. As long as we believe we can win the battle, we will be victorious to that extent.

It's about channeling our energies, our body, our mind, and our time to do one thing and, just one thing, win the battle against cancer! We must remember that if others could do it, I can do it too!

It is true that each person lives the disease differently and that we are all going to feel more or less affected than others. Still, the reality of the case is that the most common symptoms during this process can be overcome by staying in a good mood and paying little attention to worry.

Concern for what we are living will generate stress and anxiety. That will disturb our psyche, alter our energies, and produce an imbalance between how I feel and how I want to feel. As much as my illness worries me, I must not forget that everyone is working towards my healing and want me to feel my best. Therefore, worrying will only make me feel bad. So the best thing I can do to help myself is to stop thinking about my illness and start thinking about my healing!

Beyond fear, worry, anxiety, uncertainty, stress, sadness and, all the mixed feelings we may feel during this hard battle, we must know that our inner will and our faith will give us the strength to face and overcome this challenge. So, what can we do during this process? What can I do during the treatment?

WHAT TO DO DURING CHEMOTHERAPY AND RADIOTHERAPY?

Chemo and radio, as many of us know it, are treatment schemes that generate a lot of fear. Especially since we don't really know what they are and what they consist of. Most of the things we know about them are references from someone else or comments we have listened to, many of them unfounded and mostly exaggerated. But what should I do if I am to receive chemo or radio? How do I cope with this situation?

The truth is that chemotherapy and radiotherapy can be rough roads to travel. Not all of us are candidates for both treatments, as we learned in previous pages. Chemo and radio are applied to tumors located in specific sites of the colon and the rectum, and, generally, treatment regimens for colorectal cancer are well tolerated by most patients.

However, there are always side effects, and you can experience it. After all, they are very strong and powerful weapons that we use to defeat cancer.

Nevertheless, not all people suffer all the side effects, and some experience a few if they feel anything.

It is necessary to take into account that cancer cells proliferate fast. Hence their ability to affect and infiltrate the surrounding tissues. For this reason, chemotherapeutic agents are aimed at destroying these rapidly growing cells. Yet, because these drugs circulate throughout our bodies, they can also damage healthy and fast-growing cells in our bodies.

Then, it is easy to realize that the side effects and clinical alterations that we could experience depend on the damage caused to our healthy cells. Usually, those that have rapid growth or turnover such as cells of the gastrointestinal tract and hematopoietic stem cell —which produce blood in the bone marrow— or those that are in the hair follicle (hair root).

The side effects of any of the treatments can cause discomfort. However, we must understand and accept the importance of destroying cancer cells. The good news is that we can take into account that many of these effects disappear quickly once the treatment is over.

The time it takes to overcome the side effects and regain strength will vary with each of us, and it is known that this depends mainly on the will we have to move forward, live, and overcome. We understand that our recovery depends on ourselves and the attitude with which we face different physical states.

Many often get discouraged by the duration of the treatment or the side effects that they may suffer. Still, if we get sick, the most important thing is to talk with our medical team and express how we feel, what is happening to us. Our doctor can help us and recommend something that will make us feel better and in this way also our loved ones.

It is even possible that another treatment scheme can be used or to modify the hours it is administered. Even so, the only way to achieve change and improve symptoms is by communicating openly with our treating doctors. We must make sure to talk with our medical team about the side effects that could affect us, how long they could last, how serious they could be. Be prepared. And above all, when to call them if we think we need help.

Most people worry about chemotherapy, whether or not it will have side effects and, if so, how those effects will be.

We Present A Summary Of Some Of The Most Common Side Effects Caused By Chemotherapy:

Fatigue

Nausea and vomiting

Infection

Hair loss

Tendency to easily bruise and bleed

Anemia (low red blood cell counts)

Changes in appetite

Constipation

Diarrhea

Mouth, tongue and throat discomfort such as ulcers (sores) and pain when swallowing

Muscle and nerve discomfort such as numbness, tingling sensation, and pain

Changes in skin and nails, such as dryness and shift in tone

Urinary changes and kidney problems

Changes in weight

Decreased ability to concentrate and focus

Humor changes

Changes in sexual desire and function

Fertility problems

HOW TO PREPARE TO GO TO THE OPERATING ROOM?

Many of us ask ourselves: What would happen if I had to operate? What should I do if they had to operate? How should I go to the operating room? What should I take with me?

Easy, we must not do anything! Luckily for us, our doctors are excellent in the operating room, and insurance will already have everything resolved by the time we get there. Still, surely there is no way I can help them?

Of course, there is, the most important thing is to feel comfortable with ourselves and be calm and relaxed, which will significantly help our medical team before and after the intervention.

So what can we do to help? Simple, we should feel as comfortable as possible and keep in mind that everything will be fine!

We have to wear comfortable clothes, preferably very light. We can shower in the usual way. We should not eat the night before surgery unless the doctor tells us otherwise. Do not use nail paint, wear collected hair, and perhaps other recommendations that each medical team can make in a particular way.

Before going to the operating room, we must also know that surgical procedures do not always end as planned outside the operating room. Additional procedures may have to be done or even change how the operation was expected to be. Nonetheless, we should not worry, as mentioned above, our medical team is fully trained to provide us with the best treatment with the maximum benefit for us.

WILL I HAVE AN OSTOMY?

W hen talking about surgical treatments, many of the surgeries related to the colon and rectum may require an ostomy.

Usually, the surgeon's first option is to maintain the continuity of the intestine through an anastomosis, especially when it comes to cancer located in the colon. However, the possibility of an ostomy will always be in the surgeon's mind.

The truth is, although for most of us, the idea of having an ostomy or "carrying a bag in the abdomen to deposit stool" is something alarming. Still, the presence of an ostomy is not the end of the world. In fact, ostomies often serve as temporary protection for some of the surgical procedures used to treat colorectal cancer.

The ostomies, like many of the things in our lives, can be temporary or definitive. This will depend on surgical procedures necessary to eliminate the tumor or the context in which surgery occurs.

The proper care of an ostomy is simple. Having an ostomy should not significantly affect our daily lives, so: Could we work and socialize if we have an ostomy?

It takes some time to get used to an ostomy, but it doesn't mean we can't go to work, to the bank, to the movies, to a party. It does not mean that we cannot lead a full and rewarding life, although, for many people, ostomies are something little known and unpleasant.

As we learn more about how to handle them and how to care for them, we will feel more comfortable with our ostomies. However, many questions may arise as we venture to start this new stage in our lives:

Can I continue in my work?

Can I continue with my partner?

Can I use public transport?

Can I go to the park, ride a bike, go swimming?

Will you realize that I have an ostomy?

How will I feel with an ostomy?

After an ostomy, we can live our daily lives again. We can do what we like, what we are passionate about, return to all the projects we had before the ostomy. Yes, as some particular things in life, "certain conditions apply." For example, practicing some sports —like those that involve direct contact— with ostomies and can injure and/or damage it.

Can we eat anything after an ostomy? The answer is yes if we can continue to enjoy our favorite dishes.

Unless the doctor indicates otherwise, patients with ostomies can continue with their usual diet and enjoying the culinary pleasures of life. However, we should consider the consumption of foods, such as fiber, to help us form soft, large shaped stools, so we try to create a bowel habit that best suits this new lifestyle.

Some foods are more likely to cause gas, diarrhea, constipation, or incomplete digestion. But that's not why we have to stop eating them, we can simply do it when we are in our homes or somewhere else where we are comfortable.

If we don't know for sure how some foods might affect us, we can consider trying them at home, one at a time, before eating them in public. If we know how our digestion affects each food, we will be less concerned about the effects of diet. This gives us the freedom to spend more time having fun with our friends.

Another quite difficult issue is knowing if we can return to our work after an ostomy. For this, it is first necessary to take some time to recover from surgery and understand as much as possible what it means to live with an ostomy.

We can calmly return to our usual work without any problem as long as we are comfortable. A different matter would be: What if I have to do forced labor or lift a lot of weight? Although heavy work could be a complicated matter to handle, our doctor can give us the best recommendations on how to protect our ostomy and avoid complications.

The most important thing is not to let worries consume us. Returning to work can be a great way to go back to the regular routine of our lives, feel comfortable with ourselves in an environment where we can socialize pleasantly with friends.

Another aspect that may cause us enough anxiety is knowing if other people are going to know or notice that we have an ostomy. If we want to tell others or not, that we have an ostomy, is quite a personal and personal matter. Some prefer to hide this information, and others feel extremely comfortable talking about their experience and how they face this new lifestyle.

Indeed, some people will need to know about our ostomy for practical reasons. Especially if we don't have a desk or a locker at work for our stoma care supplies. In these cases, we may have to give some details to someone at work to help us with the proper arrangements and thus feel more comfortable.

On the other hand, there are many ways to "cover" an ostomy so that it is practically invisible to others. However, for us, the ostomy bag we are wearing is undeniable.

It is possible to think that every noise that comes from the ostomy is loud, and everyone around us hears them, but this is not so. Many times this feeling is only in our mind because of the shame and concern we'll have if someone finds out about our ostomy.

It is necessary to understand that most people will not know anything about our ostomy unless we tell them ourselves. Likewise, little by little, we will discover that as we get used to this new stage, we will find better ways to cope with it and feel good about ourselves and others.

It is also important to remember that if we have an ostomy, we can wear the clothes that we like the most and dress as we please. Nevertheless, we must take into account that body contour and location of the ostomy could make us feel uncomfortable with some clothes. But we must not let an ostomy limit us when dressing. It can be practical to find the ideal garments that make us look good and feel comfortable, there are even swimsuits adapted for patients with ostomies.

Although having an ostomy could make us feel uncomfortable when taking a trip or going for a walk, there are no limits to go to the places we want. Just take into account that we must take all the necessary tools to take care of our ostomy at all times, whether we travel by car, plane, train, boat, or just during a walk in the park. The limits are only set by us, not the ostomy.

Sure there are many topics that we are curious about but that many do not dare to ask. One of them is sex, the vast majority of us are thinking right now. Can I have a healthy sex life after an ostomy?

Of course, although this is a fairly broad topic to discuss in this chapter, the presence of an ostomy in our body does not prevent us from enjoying a full and rewarding sex life. We just need to get in touch with our partner and together find a way to enjoy our intimacy again. Concerning this issue, it is always good to ask our treating doctor for help and recommendations and consult with a psychologist or sexologist, they can surely help us.

An amicable way to learn to live with an ostomy is to share experiences with other people who have ostomies. This will always help us find useful and practical advice on how to manage and care for our ostomy. Finally, we might find the answer to one of the most disturbing questions of all: Will I be able to evacuate normally?

This is one of the most frequent questions in the medical consultations of patients with ostomies or candidates to have them. A terminal colostomy might indeed be for life. But many patients, with the proper training, get to create evacuation habits so regular that they do not have to change or empty their stoma bag in places other than home or office.

This peculiar pattern of adaptation to the elimination of feces through the ostomy would allow us to choose the most suitable time for the replacement or emptying of the collection bag facilitating the cleaning of the area and making us feel more comfortable by not having to do it in public or awkward places.

So, to answer the question of whether we can normally evacuate again, the answer is: it depends! If the ostomy is temporary, the intestinal transit can be restored, and for sure, we will have a regular evacuation when fulfilling the time and function for which the ostomy was created. If the ostomy is final, we have to start using the right tools to educate and care for our ostomy!

The first step is to understand that an ostomy is part of us and will accompany us wherever we go. Therefore, we must treat and care for it like any part of our body.

The next thing is to know that we can and should keep our ostomy clean and sealed to avoid bad odors and avoid bothering others. As with the rest of our body, proper grooming is vital to our healthy coexistence in society.

Another important aspect is to know that our diet directly influences our evacuation habits. In this way, a healthy diet will help us "train" and "educate" our intestines. We could somehow choose the best time to evacuate it, so as well, estimate the quantity, form, and consistency of the feces that are produced.

Finally, we must remember that the best way to use a base and bag for ostomies is with proper training by a trained health professional in the area. Professionals will give us the guidelines and recommendations necessary to optimize the duration of these devices, with adequate formation, stoma care can be done fast and efficiently by the patient.

CHAPTER V:

Living without cancer!

Many times we hear people talk about cancer as the world's greatest calamity, and as if we are all going to suffer from this disease at some point in our lives.

It is possible that, for many, cancer is a problematic word to listen to and even more, to internalize. It is very likely that for a large number of people, cancer is a frightening disease that causes great fear and concern for them.

Cancer is a painful disease to carry. But this does not mean that it is the end of the world nor the greatest calamity we can go through. It's not even true we are all going to have cancer or die from it. The only thing that is quite encouraging is that: it is possible to live without cancer!

HOW TO AVOID IT?

To avoid suffering from colorectal cancer or any other type of cancer, we need to understand it, know what it is, where it comes from, and how it occurs. The knowledge about colorectal cancer allows us to try to get it away from our body, and enjoy a long and full "cancer-free" life.

Although the possibility of "avoiding cancer" seems like taken from a futuristic movie, where if we take a daily capsule we could protect ourselves against all diseases... the idea of being able to avoid it is based on doing things that keep us away from cancer.

For example, try to modify the risk factors for this disease.

There are risk factors for colorectal cancer that can be modified and, in this way, diminish our chance of suffering from it. The detail here would be to ask:

What things can we do to prevent colorectal cancer?

How do I protect myself and my loved ones from this disease?

Is it challenging to try to modify the risk factors?

Like many things in our lives, the first thing we must have to do to achieve something is to have the will and commitment to do it! So, here we have two exciting premises that are:

Yes, it is possible to modify the risk factors and ...

No, it is not very difficult to modify the risk factors.

Constantly working on the modification of "modifiable" risk factors to prevent colorectal cancer is an excellent tool to reduce the possibility of developing this disease.

However, we must foresee that: "if something bad can happen, it will happen." That is why we should not leave everything to chance and neglect our bodies until our health is compromised.

Perhaps some people by nature, genetics, divine will, destiny, chance, bad luck, or whatever it may be going through their minds at this time, will develop colorectal cancer at some point. They will probably get it no matter what they do. Still, it is up to them to do everything possible to delay it, "preventing" this event and to act when it occurs.

WHAT DO I DO
TO AVOID IT?

When we talk about "acting" against cancer, we mean that we must detect it quickly and start working on our healing as soon as possible. This is the easiest and fastest way to ensure our victory against this disease.

Many claim that colorectal cancer is one of the easiest to detect, however, it is the least detected of all.

The methods of screening and early diagnosis are many, simple and inexpensive: from a stool or blood test to a simple rectal examination or a colonoscopy, so what can we do to prevent it? What should we do if it has not been diagnosed?

The first recommendation that any doctor would make us would be: change your lifestyle for a healthier way! The modifiable risk factors are based on what we eat, what we drink, the way we do our daily activities. In general, in the way we live "every day." But what can we do to improve this? Can I be healthier?

The answer is yes and, also, it is effortless!

Improve your diet and consume more fiber!

Fiber increases the volume of feces and absorbs water to make them softer.

Large, soft, and bulky stools move better through the colon. This allows them to be evacuated easier, that is, the fiber helps fight constipation. It helps maintain a good intestinal transit, which decreases the trauma stool generates on colon mucosa.

We must eat at least 30 grams of fiber every day. An easy way to know how much fiber is in the food we consume is by reviewing nutritional information on the food packaging, so we see the amount of fiber provided by portion.

The best sources of fiber are fruits, vegetables, and whole grains. We can eat fruits and vegetables without peeling them and choose whole fruits and vegetables instead of juices.

We can also choose bread and cereals whose packages include whole wheat, oats, or bran as the main ingredients.

Fruits, vegetables, and whole grains also contain a variety of vitamins, minerals, and antioxidants, which can influence cancer prevention. We can choose a wide range of fruits and vegetables so that we incorporate various vitamins and nutrients.

Drink water every day.

Drinking enough water, at least 2 liters a day, and other liquids in combination with fiber allow stools to be softer and more abundant. This allows for better and faster stimulation of bowel movement.

To achieve variety, we can add a touch of lemon juice to the water so that it has more flavor or, we can try other drinks that do not have gas or caffeine. Prune juice can be beneficial because it has a natural emollient effect.

We can reduce the risk of colorectal cancer by making changes in our daily lifestyle with some simple recommendations:

If you drink alcohol, do it in moderation. If we choose to drink alcohol, we should limit the amount we drink.

Stop smoking. We can talk to our doctors about the most appropriate ways to quit cigarettes. Remember, smoking alone is the most critical risk factor for colorectal cancer development.

Do exercises almost every day of the week. Exercising at least 30 minutes every day is a great way to stay healthy and active. Good daily physical activity strengthens our immune system, makes us feel more energetic, younger and capable of everything. An excellent daily walk even stimulates bowel movements!

If we are usually inactive, then we must begin to exercise. Let's start slowly and gradually to create a new and healthy habit in our bodies until we reach our goal of about 30 minutes of daily physical activity. Also, it is always good to consult with our doctors before starting an exercise program.

Maintain a healthy weight. If at this time, we have an adequate weight for our height, we must strive to maintain it. A suitable weight for us protects us from many diseases, not only cancer.

If, on the contrary, we need to lose some weight, we can quickly consult our doctor about simple healthy ways to achieve our goal. If we try to lose weight speedily and uncontrollably with aggressive programs and rigorous diets without a nutritional guide, it can be even more harmful than the same overweight.

An excellent daily combination of exercise with a balanced and healthy diet is the best tool to maintain a good weight and feel healthy and comfortable with our body.

There are several analysis options for the detection of colorectal cancer, each with advantages and disadvantages in terms of cost, discomfort, and preparation.

Get screened for colorectal cancer, people at low risk for colorectal cancer can begin screening tests at age 50. However, those at high risk, like those with family history, should start analysis sooner, even at ages like 35 years.

CHAPTER VI:

❊ ❊ ❊

Life after cancer

Is there anything after cancer?

What do these questions refer to?

What does the phrase "after cancer" really mean?

If you are diagnosed with "colon or rectal cancer," and you are treated and you are doing well: now you fully understand what it means to have a life "after cancer."

It means that after the news, after diagnosis, after asking "why me?", after surgery, chemotherapy, radiotherapy, discourage, pain, uncertainty, after the fear, the agony, the sorrows, that's where you are now.

You will realize that this can become a long time because you will take advantage of this period as you never had before!

Of course, there is something "after cancer." Cancer can be

cured and removed from our bodies, from our mind. We can be healthy, strong and independent people again, with projects and goals. Someone who wants to continue living and continue enjoying this wonderful gift that only God —or the superior intelligence that fits your beliefs— can give us, is ready to have a full and happy life to enjoy and share.

It is necessary to understand that "after cancer," there are many blessings and opportunities. It is an excellent time to consider new goals and projects. We realize life goes on, and there is no greater gift than being able to share with our loved ones, regardless of our results, our prognosis, or our life expectancy. "After cancer" is an excellent time to enjoy and share with greater passion and delivery every minute of our beautiful lives.

OVERCOMING
THE FEAR

Before starting to talk, it is necessary to sketch or define some ideas, and to begin, we must ask ourselves: "What is Fear? What is the feeling of discouragement that I have? What is the way to progress or how I think of a way to overcome it?

I must identify what I fear, what the fear is due to.

The fear of cancer?

The fear of suffering, of despair?

The fear of pain, agony, death?

The fear of having to give up our loved ones?

The fear of leaving loved ones unprotected or leaving together?

If we look in a dictionary for the definition of fear we will find something like:

"The unpleasant spiritual sensation that is translated to the body and that when manifested in the body, paralyzes us and makes us feel vulnerable and unstable."

But in reality, fear goes beyond this concept. Fear has as many definitions because each of us perceives fear in its own particular way. However, we could name the main cause of this fear as the "fear of the unknown." Many may even be afraid of what the future holds, what it could become, or what could arise with a given situation.

In the structure of time, fear is located in the future, just as pain is located in the past. Then as humans, we debate between anxiety and discomfort!

Fear is like a dark night in the middle of nowhere where we cannot see what happens around us and where there is no point of support. Now, instead of understanding, we begin to fill that space with uncertainties and dark thoughts such as: what would happen if I do this? If I stop doing that? These are thoughts that may not have an immediate response. Still, there is something that can help us: understanding fear is just fear and, and that it is necessary to understand it, face it, explore it so we will be able to defeat it. Then why fight to overcome fear if we can set out to understand and learn, rather than to control it, to live in your company?

Fear, like many other things, arises from ignorance, restlessness, uncertainty. So only by knowing where anxiety comes from, we can try to understand fear, live with it, and overcome it.

Living without fear is impossible. Nobody is safe or beyond doubt, and, in this case, the fear of pain, suffering, or death will always be present. Also, how can we run faster, be more agile, and fight harder against a disease without the most significant impulse of the human spirit that is the fear of death? If we fight against something, we must fight against the greatest evil of all, represented by indifference, laziness, lack of compassion, and brotherhood with others. So what is wrong with being afraid? Why do we fear so many things?

We can feel a great fear of death, of not being with our loved ones, of not walking on this earth, but as we can see, fear, like many other feelings, is absolutely necessary. However, it is also essential to learn to understand it, to handle it, and to live in harmony with it. We need to learn to use fear as an ally and not as an enemy. Fear gives us that high impulse to not abandon chemotherapy, to continue attending radiotherapy, to accept surgery, to promptly go to the control check-ups. And that fear will be the same that drives us and helps us survive and overcome the disease.

If we understand that maintaining a healthy lifestyle, a balanced life, if we go to the doctor regularly, accept help to continue and recover our health, take the medications, attend the necessary therapies, and if we decide to understand cancer, we will have the best of opportunities. We will be able to defeat this disease.

This victory, entirely achievable, will allow us to continue maintaining a full and rewarding life alongside our loved ones.

So, the only question we should really ask ourselves is:

Why be afraid of cancer?

UNDERSTANDING CANCER

If for some reason, we had a fear of hearing unfavorable things or we are facing different emotions than usual, we could carry out this task by having a person next to us. Someone who could accompany us and hold hands while confronting these experiences. Either a close and trustworthy person or merely a therapist with expertise in the area.

Cancer, as a disease, generates a deep fear in any of us. It is something new but harmful that will lead us to travel a path of uncertainty, pain, worries, and hopelessness.

Especially if we are poorly informed about its nature, and if we isolate ourselves and refuse to get help to deal with this situation.

However, the most important thing about this situation is to understand what is happening.

For this, it is necessary to understand that all the results we obtain depend on the decisions we make on the paths that we decided to travel, how is that possible?

Clinical Psychoneuroimmunology appeared about 40 years ago when two American scientists, Robert Ader (psychologist) and Nicholas Cohen (immunologist), surprised the scientific community by demonstrating through their scientific experiments in rats how a nervous stimulus altered the cells of the immune system.

This exciting science began its first steps offering the opportunity to discover the interaction between the nervous system and the immune system. Focusing on our nervous system as a channel capable of translating feelings into biochemical substances, among many other functions, it can generate a change in the production and function of lymphocytes, neutrophils, and natural killer cells. Tissue infection or inflammation can predispose us to have certain attitudes in life due to the production of cytokines, which function as messengers communicating to the brain how the organs in your body are working.

Imagine what it meant: the fact of being able to discover through science how intestinal flora decreases the chances of suffering from diseases such as depression, autoimmune pathologies, hormonal problems, fibromyalgia, and other symptoms.

As scientist Leo Pruimboom says, "psychoneuroimmunology answers the question why." This science studies the mechanism of action of disease or pain.

The therapist or doctor has more tools to be able to make a more complete diagnosis, and thus be able to help the person from a more comprehensive point of view.

By knowing the pathophysiology of the disease is easier to approach the possible origins that are causing a particular health problem.

You can save yourself excessive amounts of medications that could cause some side effects. Knowing the mechanism of action allows you to be more specific in the treatment and use the medication that is most suitable to help you.

The mechanism of action and the use of the therapies proposed in psychoneuroimmunology are carried out through outstanding scientific support. Because science is the mechanism we have in today's society to get as close as possible to the truth and achieve the maximum possible agreement between the scientific community and society.

Psychoneuroimmunology integrates the body as a set of interactions where a stimulus can affect all the systems of the body.

Another characteristic that makes psychoneuroimmunology unique is the consideration that there is an environment that can affect the person's perception of their disease. The doctors and therapists who are dedicated to this science know how horrifying they can be, specific names of diseases elegantly called "labels." Currently, many medications are spent to alleviate the side effects of chronic diseases that they say have no solution.

This would be an essential point to discuss. It means one thing not to know the origin that causes this disease and another very different thinking there is no solution.

No human being wants to suffer nor wants someone else to suffer. Therefore, the best thing we have to do to face cancer is understanding it. We have to learn about it and how to handle this terrible disease.

Colon and rectal cancer develop slowly, and it takes many years for the inflamed cells to become premalignant, and these become malignant tumors or cancer itself. Therefore, prevention and regular doctor visits can help us reduce mortality due to this disease. This means that it is indispensable to understand that following the recommendations given by the health expert personnel on the management of this pathology is essential to keep us healthy and away from this latent danger.

Likewise, our ability to understand and help in these matters will go hand in hand with our willingness to learn about the disease, and also how we transmit this knowledge to others. Because only in this way can we contribute positively to our health and that of anyone who needs it.

HELPING UNDERSTAND CANCER

The only way to help understand how eventualities and situations that may arise are handled is to learn to understand it first ourselves. It is impossible to try to teach other people or to help others if we are not able to help us first.

Only by learning to face our internal struggle and learning to overcome our fears will we be able to be a source of support, help, strength, and hope for our loved ones and those around us.

If any of us has been a cancer patient, then this section will be like walking a path already known. If, on the contrary, we have never suffered from this disease, then we have much to learn about it. We have to teach and accompany other people transmitting the idea that there are many things beyond cancer.

First of all, we need to understand every who suffers from cancer is a sensitive person, and with an accentuated level of anguish. It's like being caught in deep uncertainty and terrible fear. A fear that even goes beyond its understanding and its own essence. It's a fear whose origin is even greater than the fear of death itself. It is a terrible fear of suffering, being unable to withstand treatments, or also not being able to receive any treatment. But above all, it is a terrible fear of abandoning your loved ones.

To be able to support a cancer patient, the only thing that matters is the love and understanding that we can provide beyond the economic and social support we have to offer. Let us remember and keep in mind the idea that a person who feels loved is a person who finds the necessary strength to fight and overcome any obstacle. Love is the greatest feeling of hope and strength that we can transmit to another human being. It is the only thing that will always have a positive effect on peace and hope in each and every one of us.

If we really want to teach other people to understand cancer, we just have to sit next to them, ask them and tell them, with real interest, how do you feel? I'm here for you!

Only in this way can we understand who we are dealing with and how much support and solidarity he needs. It is necessary they unequivocally perceive that they are not alone, that there is a full and happy life beyond this disease.

As friends or family, we could start by transmitting what we think and what we have learned. But also, with all the love we have. So that they do not feel that we give any bad news. We must remember that bad news does not exist. They are only news and, depending on the way we transmit them, we can positively or negatively influence others.

We can also offer a helping hand and a point of support when you go to the doctor's office or to the administration of the treatments. It is vital to make them feel that they are not alone and that they can always count on our support and company.

Likewise, it is good to recommend a book or to read material containing relevant information about the disease. None of us like the idea of starting to learn about something that is affecting us, and that is harmful to us. The only way to understand what we go through is by understanding the disease and how to deal with it.

CHAPTER VII:

* * *

Some Tips

WHAT CAN I EAT?

An interesting question with a great answer is that we all simply rejoice when they tell us: you can eat everything! Little phrases indeed make life happy in many ways, it is lovely to feel free to eat everything!

The freedom to eat literally "anything" is the same freedom we should feel when doing "anything." Having cancer does not mean we stop being ourselves. On the contrary, we have to try to be happier and feel freer than ever because we are struggling with a fierce enemy whom we know we can defeat and learn a lot from.But are there any foods better than others? Are there foods that make us feel better than others? Are there times to eat a particular kind of food?

One food is really no better than another. The most important thing is to add fiber-containing foods to our daily diet and drink lots of fluids, as mentioned in Chapter V.
Fiber and water as companions of a healthy and balanced diet will help us, above all, to maintain proper intestinal transit and to have soft stools. This is very important so that they do not cause discomfort or bleeding at the time of having contact with the tumor during the evacuation, especially if the cancer is in the rectum.

As general recommendations, we should avoid foods that cause us gastrointestinal discomfort or that are not very appealing to us. Otherwise, we can eat everything we want and make us happy!

Now, what can I eat if I should have surgery? Before surgery, it is not necessary to have any particular diet unless our medical team indicates otherwise. Special considerations are made the day before the operation, and, for this, the medical team will give us all the recommendations to follow.

During the postoperative period, the story is different. At this stage, the food we can consume will gradually increase consistency according to the indications of the surgical team until all the necessary and adequate nutrients for an ostomy or anastomosis are ingested.

Postoperative recommendations depend in no small extent on each surgical group and the experience they have with one or another food. However, we must remember that, after passing a gradual recovery process, we can once again eat "everything we like."

After surgery, we become ourselves again. Beyond some simple recommendations, we can eat almost everything again, as long as these foods do not cause gastrointestinal problems.

In the case that we get an ostomy, it is advisable to maintain a certain degree of "constipation." In these cases, remember that we can eat and drink everything we like as before surgery, but we must try to avoid foods that soften stool or produce gas.

In general, the only objection to food would be the discomfort caused by irregular bowel movements or the production of many gases, but this is something that patients can regulate.

WHAT EXERCISES AND PHYSICAL ACTIVITIES CAN I DO AFTER SURGERY?

We all know the beneficial effects of physical activity: the release endorphins, improve circulation, breathing, mood, and even decrease the sensation of pain.

For all this, getting moving as soon as possible helps us recover faster!

In the first months after surgery, the abdomen will be recovering from its wounds, and the fear of presenting a hernia or eventration will be present. However, by limiting the force applied directly to the scar or using an abdominal belt we can reduce the risks.

There are no limitations to live a full life after surgery. All we have to remember is to protect ourselves a little more when performing vigorous exercises or contact activities such as practicing martial arts.

However, specific questions will inevitably arise. Such as: Can I exercise if I have an ostomy?, or can I swim if I have an ostomy?, or what exercises can I do if I have an ostomy?

Of course, we do! Of course we can exercise if we have an ostomy. However, we must take into account some considerations.

Having an ostomy makes it easier to become dehydrated, so drinking lots of water is essential. It is also important to eat some carbohydrates before starting the activities, these will help to absorb water better and give us energy.

The most important thing is to listen to and know our bodies. If something hurts, stop. If any activity is very exhausting or demanding for us, we must decrease the intensity. We will recover all our physical strength gradually, and we will be able to carry out the activities we had used and even many more.

It is essential to feel comfortable when deciding what kind of physical activity to perform. Especially if we feel any discomfort concerning showing ourselves in public with an ostomy. Today there are exclusive one-piece or high-cut swimsuits —in the case of women— or sports shirts to cover the torso in men. Even with the right conditions, swimming with an ostomy can be a great way to exercise, relax, and share with family and friends.

HERE ARE SOME QUESTIONS TO WHICH WE SHOULD HAVE ANSWERS BEFORE SURGERY:

The following list shows the most frequently asked questions that we should keep in mind when consulting with the medical and surgical team. They will help us solve many doubts and feel more secure:

What doctor, medical group, or hospital should I choose?How do I choose it? Who decides it: a relative or me? What do I rely on for this election?

Why should I have surgery?

How will they operate on me?

Are there any other options? Is this the best for me?

What are the risks of this surgery?

Will the colon be sutured, or do I need the training to take care of an ostomy?

What will anesthesia be like?

What should I do before surgery?

Should I change my diet before?

How much an I eat before and after surgery?

Should I take any medication or stop any that I already take?

Will I take medication after surgery?

How much pain will I feel after surgery?

For what daily activities will I need help after surgery?

When can I return to my normal activities?

What can I do to feel better?

Do you have any other questions?

TIPS FOR MANAGING POSTOPERATIVE WOUNDS:

How to care for and heal them.

It is essential to follow the recommendations of the medical team.

To Remove The Dressings (Gauze And Adhesives) That Cover The Wound Before Showering Or Changing Them, We Must:

Wash our hands with soap and water for 15-30 seconds.
Gently remove the adhesive and gauze and discard them in the trash, we can wear gloves to do this.

To Wash The Wound In The Shower:

We can take a shower sitting or standing, with warm water or at room temperature.

We should not dive into the bathtub until the stitches, sutures, or staples are removed.

Shower for about 5 to 10 minutes, keeping the wound out of the direct impact of the water.

With gentleness and a little pressure, try to remove clots or fluid accumulated under the skin.

Keep the friction of the wound to a minimum.

To Clean The Wound Outside The Shower:

Choose a clean area to discover the wound.

The cleanest area should be the most covered, the area of the sutures or staples, so we will start cleaning around it.

With a soft gauze impregnated in saline solution, sterile water, soapy solution, or the doctor's recommendation, try to remove clots or secretion with a gentle movement of pressure on the wound.

To Cover The Wound After Cleaning It:

We can wear gloves and place the gauze to cover so that it slightly exceeds the edges of the wound, so we protect a little more from contamination.

We must keep the wound clean, dry, and covered with adhesive to prevent the entry of contaminants or moisture.

WHEN TO CONTACT YOUR DOCTOR OR COLOPROCTOLOGIST AHEAD OF SCHEDULE?

We should contact our doctor or coloproctologist as soon as possible [or right away] if we are presented with:

Incessant pain
Pain that gets worse
Fever
Nausea or lack of appetite
Continuous vomiting
Redness, pain, or foul-smelling discharge through the wound
Bleeding
Changes in the color or size of the ostomy (if we have it)
Increase in volume in the abdomen
Several days without bowel movements after surgery

"HEALING THE BODY"

Carmen Esther López

Emotions, thoughts, have manifestations in the body.

This means that all those emotions of fear, anger, resentment, deep pain of the past, finding no meaning in life or the world. Any thought and feeling that comes from a loss or lack, that lasts over time or which has an impact on us, are extreme and also, abrupt, and can take a toll on our health.

From the scientific point of view, the above has been demonstrated. So, in addition to the treatment that we must perform on the physical body (surgery, chemotherapy, radiotherapy), we must also carry out treatment of our mind and emotions.

This treatment must be sincere and real, from the authenticity of being ourselves, with absolute certainty and confidence, without fears.

Authenticity in the purification of thoughts and emotions is what will manifest itself in the healing of the physical body. For this debugging, we need to be alert in the thinking we have. Many times it is not easy to find that thought (sometimes it hides behind many other beliefs). Still, one way of observing and being alert to feelings is when we have an emotion that generates uneasiness, lack of peace. Let's go to the thought that's making it, and that is where we have to act.

How can we act? Changing that thought that generates pain, anger, loneliness, fear, from lack of liberation from the past. This "treatment" of the mind or thought process will depend solely on you, that is to say, the state of alertness to which you are willing to improve is the way through which you reach healing.

Our thoughts are energy, this energy is projected and has a manifestation. By changing this energy, we alter that projection. And therefore, the physical expression since it is another thought that is being projected.

This thought or emotion that causes restlessness and lack of peace is generally repetitive. We are attached to that thought (without realizing it) and do not let go. For example: because we believe we are right (in some event of our lives) and that's why we do not give in. We become more rooted in that thought. That's the thought we must change for a better one.

That other thought must be pure, real, sincere, of peace, of fullness, that takes us out of the pit of pessimism, of victimhood, arrogance, of the non-acceptance of day-to-day events, of hostility. It has to be a liberating thought of all the bonds created by your thoughts. That feeling was making you suffer, either for losses or deficiencies. Opinions you wrongly believed were indispensable for your life. By becoming aware that "it" is not essential for your life, then you'll "release" all those bonds you created. Obligations towards people, things, unreached goals, etc. You create a different atmosphere of peace and harmony in your being. You realize the lack of importance that "it" has for your life, so you can live without "it."

In this way, mind change begins, so change on surrounding events begins, because it is a change of energy emitted and perceived by thoughts.

"YOU ARE NOT A DIAGNOSIS"

Priest Gabriel Flores

I wanted to give continuity to the review by Dr. Carmen Esther, entitling this text: "Healing the spirit." But I have always liked the expression: "You are not a diagnosis." As a priest, I have felt in the first person the limited experiences of the human being, the joy of being born, experiences of growth, psycho-affective crises, questions of the man with God, agony, and death, among many others...

Life is a progressive experience that makes us cling to it, in its different tastes, people, situations, status. The circumstances of life affect us, transform us, and make us who we are, indeed. But I firmly believe that this does not define us completely. Life is that constant longing to want to wake up, but how hard it is when we have to face a diagnosis? To say: "I was diagnosed with cancer". Yes, it is terrifying. The world and dreams begin to fall apart little by little. It seems that we are beginning to understand what many things mean at the moment they give us the "diagnosis." I believe a diagnosis does NOT define us, you are NOT what you have, you are not a disease... You are life. And even though what you are going through can be a consequence of multiple physiological or genetic aspects, maybe everything could be different if we all had an education that built us more human and spiritually.

But we don't. As we grow, we become aware of our spirit, maybe by the influence of friends, life lessons, mistakes, falls and rises...

or books like this.

I insist, a diagnosis does not make us, does not condemn us, does not threaten us. How nice is that this text can be an instrument to give us that information, help us to overcome fear and make us responsible for our health. A diagnosis is not the end.

Another situation that, without a doubt, also takes us to the limit is the issue of "modesty." Why talk about modesty and cancer? Because right there, at the time of diagnosis, a new life also begins. When "I no longer have privacy." I have to fight against my pain, the nakedness of my body becomes a medical work area. I even end up feeling that I may lose my dignity. It is time to accept our body as it is, and now with a disease. It is precisely in these topics where we must arm ourselves with strength. When we must realize that our life and our body need not to be a cause of shame. Perhaps society and its hypersexualized culture have led us to these ideals of perfection. But when you accept yourself and realize that we are all equal, and at the end of the day, we are just a body that is neither good nor bad. A body God made, and that He has a clear purpose for and who is undoubtedly putting everything in his hands.

Knowing this, let us initiate an act of faith in yourself and in your doctors. You do not have to fear judgment. Your health is worth more than beliefs and mental barriers that we sometimes have, so cheer up!

As a man of faith, I genuinely believe that we are in this world for a purpose, after all, the question "why me?", "Why do I have to suffer?" those are always necessary, and still have answers. I want you to know that "God does everything well." In the book of Genesis, we are told that we are his most perfect work, his image and likeness, an extension of his love for the world so we could sustain his creation and all creatures. Not only that, later they tell us about a man in Nazareth who gave his life for you or me. A man who had no other way than suffering to achieve salvation for men, and who was hung naked on a cross. Knowing this leads me to understand that I am not alone, that Christ overcame many things for me, and that I can do beautiful things too. I can contribute with something so that everything that God has done can return to him and reach its fullness. Thinking of a goal: peace, love, heaven, helps me understand that I am here for something and that nothing returns without bearing fruit. Like the rain... that leaves fertile land in its wake and renews life in nature.

So, using these perceptions to turn my diagnosis into an act of faith, confidence flourishes in me: I can overcome this, I can get ahead. God is stronger than the disease. This critical moment in my life propels me to transcend. In essence, through prayer and meditation, I obtain almost half of my healing because my peace does not come from material things. I dare to say, not even from the body... my peace comes from God.

I saw a child die at birth, had no diagnosis, had no time to wander, fall, or get up. Living that experience was very painful personally, what can I say to his mother who waited for him with great enthusiasm for 9 months? No,

I felt the pain of not being able to say anything, only offer my silence and company. Crying is allowed, the opportune hug and the faithful prayer. If God is good, why does that happen? It is difficult to understand God's purposes. However, this little boy teaches us not to be petty, to value our lives, to continue living it, to fulfill treatment without hesitation, to know that we do not need a positive or negative result. To understand that our life is sustained by God.

Think about this:

Who of you by worrying can add a single hour to your life? Since you cannot do this very little thing, why do you worry about the rest? Consider how the wildflowers grow. They do not labor or spin. Yet I tell you, not even Solomon in all his splendor was dressed like one of these. If that is how God clothes the grass of the field, which is here today, and tomorrow is thrown into the fire, how much more will he take care of you—you of little faith!" Lk. 12,27-28.

From faith, everything is more bearable. A friend of only 10 years who survived cancer and never stopped smiling, always said: "Smiling heals," "Singing heals" and clung deeply to God. The healing process is not just for treating cancer, it is your whole life. Dare to live the experience of God, and even if there are no exits, and although this life hurts, you will realize that God is stronger. In the Word of God, in the book of Isaiah. 41.10 says:

"Do not fear because I am with you, do not be distressed, because I am your God, I will strengthen you, and I will help you, I will support you with my victorious Right Hand."

Definitely:

You are not a diagnosis... God is stronger.

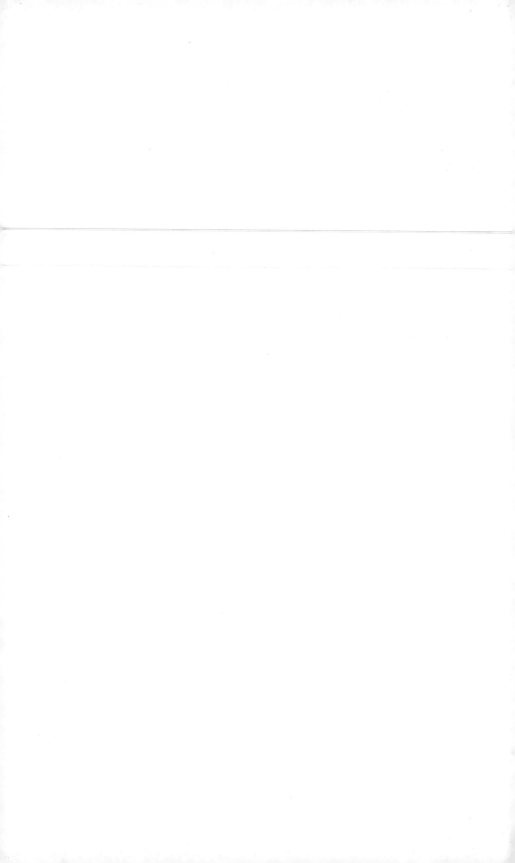

Printed in Great Britain
by Amazon

60132568R00068